If there is effort, there is always accomplishment.

- Jigoro Kano

© Copyright 2014 Randy T. Olson

All rights reserved. No part of this book may be
reproduced in any form without written permission
from the publisher.

Published through Amazon.com
ISBN-13: 978-1500875206

Index

Forward _____ 5

Patient Information _____ 7
   Patient name, address and phone number
   Care-person
   Type of surgery
   Drug allergies
   Insurance Company
   Policy number
   Insurance Company and phone number
   Doctor name and phone number
   Emergency room phone number

Doctor, Specialist and Assistant Information _____ 9
   Name, address and phone number

Daily Medication and Statistics Charts _____ 11-79
   Medication names
   Doses and when taken
   Weight
   Temperature
   Hour's slept
   Heart rate
   Wellness gage
   Notes

Calendar's _____ 81-89
   2014 through 2018 and appointments

Forward

Having gone through open heart surgery I was unable to remember what or when I had taken a pill, what my health statistics were or what was going on with my recovery. My sister generously took time to create a book of forms so I could write down what I was doing. Thank goodness she did! I have elaborated on her idea and created a concise collection of forms which all post-surgery patients can easily document the basic aspects of recovery.

This diary is for all out-patients who want to take charge of daily medication, activity and healing process. Each day offers a visual account of your progress from one day to the next. It also offers clear and precise charts for doctors to see how far you have come in your recovery.

Take time each day to track and document your progress. You will be surprised at what transpires day by day over a one month period. Family members, who offer their assistance, will find this to be a valuable aid in your healing. Their addition to your chart is necessary when you are unable to do it for yourself.

Using this **Post Surgery Recovery Diary** you will never have trouble medicating or guessing what has occurred during your recuperation when everything is documented.

All my best to your successful recovery,
Randy T. Olson

Patient Information

Patient name_____

Address_____

Date of birth_____

City and State of birth_____

Phone number_____

Care-person_____

Address_____

Phone number_____

Type of surgery_____

Drug allergies_____

Insurance Company_____

Policy number_____

Phone number_____

Doctor_____

Doctor phone number_____

Hospital emergency phone number_____

Doctor, Assistant and Specialist Information

Name_____
Address_____
Phone number_____

Name_____
Address_____
Phone number_____

Name_____
Address_____
Phone number_____

Name_____
Address_____
Phone number_____

Name_____
Address_____
Phone number_____

Name_____
Address_____
Phone number_____

Name_____
Address_____
Phone number_____

Name_____
Address_____
Phone number_____

Notes

Daily Medication

Date ____/____/____

Medications	Morning	Afternoon	Evening
Drug & Dose:	Time:		
Drug & Dose:			
Drug & Dose:			
Drug & Dose:			
Drug & Dose:			
Drug & Dose:			
Drug & Dose:			

Daily Statistics

Weight:	Temp:	Hours Slept:
Heart rate:	Walking time:	Blood Pressure:
How do you feel (1 being poor) circle:	1 2 3 4 5 6 7 8 9 10	

Notes

Daily Medication

Date ____/____/____

Medications	Morning	Afternoon	Evening
Drug & Dose:	Time:		
Drug & Dose:			
Drug & Dose:			
Drug & Dose:			
Drug & Dose:			
Drug & Dose:			
Drug & Dose:			

Daily Statistics

Weight:	Temp:	Hours Slept:
Heart rate:	Walking time:	Blood Pressure:
How do you feel ⇨ (1 being poor) circle:	1 2 3 4 5 6 7 8 9 10	

Notes

Daily Medication

Date ____/____/____

Medications	Morning	Afternoon	Evening
Drug & Dose:	Time:		
Drug & Dose:			
Drug & Dose:			
Drug & Dose:			
Drug & Dose:			
Drug & Dose:			
Drug & Dose:			

Daily Statistics

Weight:	Temp:	Hours Slept:
Heart rate:	Walking time:	Blood Pressure:
How do you feel ⇨ (1 being poor) circle:	1 2 3 4 5 6 7 8 9 10	

Notes

Daily Medication

Date ____/____/____

Medications	Morning	Afternoon	Evening
Drug & Dose:	Time:		
Drug & Dose:			
Drug & Dose:			
Drug & Dose:			
Drug & Dose:			
Drug & Dose:			
Drug & Dose:			

Daily Statistics

Weight:	Temp:	Hours Slept:
Heart rate:	Walking time:	Blood Pressure:
How do you feel ⇨ (1 being poor) circle:	1 2 3 4 5 6 7 8 9 10	

Notes

Daily Medication

Date ____/____/____

Medications	Morning	Afternoon	Evening
Drug & Dose:	Time:		
Drug & Dose:			
Drug & Dose:			
Drug & Dose:			
Drug & Dose:			
Drug & Dose:			
Drug & Dose:			

Daily Statistics

Weight:	Temp:	Hours Slept:
Heart rate:	Walking time:	Blood Pressure:
How do you feel ⇒ (1 being poor) circle:	1 2 3 4 5 6 7 8 9 10	

Notes

Daily Medication

Date ____/____/____

Medications	Morning	Afternoon	Evening
Drug & Dose:	Time:		
Drug & Dose:			
Drug & Dose:			
Drug & Dose:			
Drug & Dose:			
Drug & Dose:			
Drug & Dose:			

Daily Statistics

Weight:	Temp:	Hours Slept:
Heart rate:	Walking time:	Blood Pressure:
How do you feel ⇨ (1 being poor) circle:	1 2 3 4 5 6 7 8 9 10	

Notes

Daily Medication

Date ____/____/____

Medications	Morning	Afternoon	Evening
Drug & Dose:	Time:		
Drug & Dose:			
Drug & Dose:			
Drug & Dose:			
Drug & Dose:			
Drug & Dose:			
Drug & Dose:			

Daily Statistics

Weight:	Temp:	Hours Slept:
Heart rate:	Walking time:	Blood Pressure:
How do you feel ⇨ (1 being poor) circle:	1 2 3 4 5 6 7 8 9 10	

Notes

Daily Medication

Date ____/____/____

Medications	Morning	Afternoon	Evening
Drug & Dose:	Time:		
Drug & Dose:			
Drug & Dose:			
Drug & Dose:			
Drug & Dose:			
Drug & Dose:			
Drug & Dose:			

Daily Statistics

Weight:	Temp:	Hours Slept:
Heart rate:	Walking time:	Blood Pressure:
How do you feel ⇨ (1 being poor) circle:	1 2 3 4 5 6 7 8 9 10	

Notes

Daily Medication

Date ____/____/____

Medications	Morning	Afternoon	Evening
Drug & Dose:	Time:		
Drug & Dose:			
Drug & Dose:			
Drug & Dose:			
Drug & Dose:			
Drug & Dose:			
Drug & Dose:			

Daily Statistics

Weight:	Temp:		Hours Slept:	
Heart rate:	Walking time:		Blood Pressure:	
How do you feel ⇨ (1 being poor) circle:	1 2 3 4 5 6 7 8 9 10			

Notes

Daily Medication

Date ____/____/____

Medications	Morning	Afternoon	Evening
Drug & Dose:	Time:		
Drug & Dose:			
Drug & Dose:			
Drug & Dose:			
Drug & Dose:			
Drug & Dose:			
Drug & Dose:			

Daily Statistics

Weight:	Temp:	Hours Slept:
Heart rate:	Walking time:	Blood Pressure:
How do you feel ⇒ (1 being poor) circle:	1 2 3 4 5 6 7 8 9 10	

Notes

Daily Medication

Date ____/____/____

Medications	Morning	Afternoon	Evening
Drug & Dose:	Time:		
Drug & Dose:			
Drug & Dose:			
Drug & Dose:			
Drug & Dose:			
Drug & Dose:			
Drug & Dose:			

Daily Statistics

Weight:	Temp:	Hours Slept:
Heart rate:	Walking time:	Blood Pressure:
How do you feel ⇨ (1 being poor) circle:	1 2 3 4 5 6 7 8 9 10	

Notes

Daily Medication

Date ____/____/____

Medications	Morning	Afternoon	Evening
Drug & Dose:	Time:		
Drug & Dose:			
Drug & Dose:			
Drug & Dose:			
Drug & Dose:			
Drug & Dose:			
Drug & Dose:			

Daily Statistics

Weight:	Temp:	Hours Slept:
Heart rate:	Walking time:	Blood Pressure:
How do you feel ⇨ (1 being poor) circle:	1 2 3 4 5 6 7 8 9 10	

Notes

Daily Medication

Date ____/____/____

Medications	Morning	Afternoon	Evening
Drug & Dose:	Time:		
Drug & Dose:			
Drug & Dose:			
Drug & Dose:			
Drug & Dose:			
Drug & Dose:			
Drug & Dose:			

Daily Statistics

Weight:	Temp:	Hours Slept:
Heart rate:	Walking time:	Blood Pressure:
How do you feel ⇨ (1 being poor) circle:	1 2 3 4 5 6 7 8 9 10	

Notes

Daily Medication

Date ____/____/____

Medications	Morning	Afternoon	Evening
Drug & Dose:	Time:		
Drug & Dose:			
Drug & Dose:			
Drug & Dose:			
Drug & Dose:			
Drug & Dose:			
Drug & Dose:			

Daily Statistics

Weight:	Temp:	Hours Slept:
Heart rate:	Walking time:	Blood Pressure:
How do you feel ⇨ (1 being poor) circle:	1 2 3 4 5 6 7 8 9 10	

Notes

Daily Medication

Date ____/____/____

Medications	Morning	Afternoon	Evening
Drug & Dose:	Time:		
Drug & Dose:			
Drug & Dose:			
Drug & Dose:			
Drug & Dose:			
Drug & Dose:			
Drug & Dose:			

Daily Statistics

Weight:	Temp:	Hours Slept:
Heart rate:	Walking time:	Blood Pressure:
How do you feel ⇨ (1 being poor) circle:	1 2 3 4 5 6 7 8 9 10	

Notes

Daily Medication

Date ____/____/____

Medications	Morning	Afternoon	Evening
Drug & Dose:	Time:		
Drug & Dose:			
Drug & Dose:			
Drug & Dose:			
Drug & Dose:			
Drug & Dose:			
Drug & Dose:			

Daily Statistics

Weight:	Temp:	Hours Slept:
Heart rate:	Walking time:	Blood Pressure:
How do you feel ⇒ (1 being poor) circle:	1 2 3 4 5 6 7 8 9 10	

Notes

Daily Medication

Date ____/____/____

Medications	Morning	Afternoon	Evening
Drug & Dose:	Time:		
Drug & Dose:			
Drug & Dose:			
Drug & Dose:			
Drug & Dose:			
Drug & Dose:			
Drug & Dose:			

Daily Statistics

Weight:	Temp:	Hours Slept:
Heart rate:	Walking time:	Blood Pressure:
How do you feel ⇨ (1 being poor) circle:	1 2 3 4 5 6 7 8 9 10	

Notes

Daily Medication

Date ____/____/____

Medications	Morning	Afternoon	Evening
Drug & Dose:	Time:		
Drug & Dose:			
Drug & Dose:			
Drug & Dose:			
Drug & Dose:			
Drug & Dose:			
Drug & Dose:			

Daily Statistics

Weight:	Temp:	Hours Slept:
Heart rate:	Walking time:	Blood Pressure:
How do you feel ⇨ (1 being poor) circle:	1 2 3 4 5 6 7 8 9 10	

Notes

Daily Medication

Date ____/____/____

Medications	Morning	Afternoon	Evening
Drug & Dose:	Time:		
Drug & Dose:			
Drug & Dose:			
Drug & Dose:			
Drug & Dose:			
Drug & Dose:			
Drug & Dose:			

Daily Statistics

Weight:	Temp:	Hours Slept:
Heart rate:	Walking time:	Blood Pressure:
How do you feel ⇨ (1 being poor) circle:	1 2 3 4 5 6 7 8 9 10	

Notes

Daily Medication

Date ____/____/____

Medications	Morning	Afternoon	Evening
Drug & Dose:	Time:		
Drug & Dose:			
Drug & Dose:			
Drug & Dose:			
Drug & Dose:			
Drug & Dose:			
Drug & Dose:			

Daily Statistics

Weight:	Temp:	Hours Slept:
Heart rate:	Walking time:	Blood Pressure:
How do you feel ⇒ (1 being poor) circle:	1 2 3 4 5 6 7 8 9 10	

Notes

Daily Medication

Date ____/____/____

Medications	Morning	Afternoon	Evening
Drug & Dose:	Time:		
Drug & Dose:			
Drug & Dose:			
Drug & Dose:			
Drug & Dose:			
Drug & Dose:			
Drug & Dose:			

Daily Statistics

Weight:	Temp:	Hours Slept:
Heart rate:	Walking time:	Blood Pressure:
How do you feel ⇨ (1 being poor) circle:	1 2 3 4 5 6 7 8 9 10	

Notes

Daily Medication

Date ____/____/____

Medications	Morning	Afternoon	Evening
Drug & Dose:	Time:		
Drug & Dose:			
Drug & Dose:			
Drug & Dose:			
Drug & Dose:			
Drug & Dose:			
Drug & Dose:			

Daily Statistics

Weight:	Temp:	Hours Slept:
Heart rate:	Walking time:	Blood Pressure:
How do you feel ⇨ (1 being poor) circle:	1 2 3 4 5 6 7 8 9 10	

Notes

Daily Medication

Date ____/____/____

Medications	Morning	Afternoon	Evening
Drug & Dose:	Time:		
Drug & Dose:			
Drug & Dose:			
Drug & Dose:			
Drug & Dose:			
Drug & Dose:			
Drug & Dose:			

Daily Statistics

Weight:	Temp:	Hours Slept:
Heart rate:	Walking time:	Blood Pressure:
How do you feel ⇨ (1 being poor) circle:	1 2 3 4 5 6 7 8 9 10	

Notes

Daily Medication

Date ____/____/____

Medications	Morning	Afternoon	Evening
Drug & Dose:	Time:		
Drug & Dose:			
Drug & Dose:			
Drug & Dose:			
Drug & Dose:			
Drug & Dose:			
Drug & Dose:			

Daily Statistics

Weight:	Temp:	Hours Slept:
Heart rate:	Walking time:	Blood Pressure:
How do you feel ⇒ (1 being poor) circle:	1 2 3 4 5 6 7 8 9 10	

Notes

Daily Medication

Date ____/____/____

Medications	Morning	Afternoon	Evening
Drug & Dose:	Time:		
Drug & Dose:			
Drug & Dose:			
Drug & Dose:			
Drug & Dose:			
Drug & Dose:			
Drug & Dose:			

Daily Statistics

Weight:	Temp:	Hours Slept:
Heart rate:	Walking time:	Blood Pressure:
How do you feel ⇨ (1 being poor) circle:	1 2 3 4 5 6 7 8 9 10	

Notes

Daily Medication

Date ____/____/____

Medications	Morning	Afternoon	Evening
Drug & Dose:	Time:		
Drug & Dose:			
Drug & Dose:			
Drug & Dose:			
Drug & Dose:			
Drug & Dose:			
Drug & Dose:			

Daily Statistics

Weight:	Temp:	Hours Slept:
Heart rate:	Walking time:	Blood Pressure:
How do you feel ⇨ (1 being poor) circle:	1 2 3 4 5 6 7 8 9 10	

Notes

Daily Medication

Date ____/____/____

Medications	Morning	Afternoon	Evening
Drug & Dose:	Time:		
Drug & Dose:			
Drug & Dose:			
Drug & Dose:			
Drug & Dose:			
Drug & Dose:			
Drug & Dose:			

Daily Statistics

Weight:	Temp:	Hours Slept:
Heart rate:	Walking time:	Blood Pressure:
How do you feel ⇨ (1 being poor) circle:	1 2 3 4 5 6 7 8 9 10	

Notes

Daily Medication

Date ____/____/____

Medications	Morning	Afternoon	Evening
Drug & Dose:	Time:		
Drug & Dose:			
Drug & Dose:			
Drug & Dose:			
Drug & Dose:			
Drug & Dose:			
Drug & Dose:			

Daily Statistics

Weight:	Temp:	Hours Slept:
Heart rate:	Walking time:	Blood Pressure:
How do you feel ⇨ (1 being poor) circle:	1 2 3 4 5 6 7 8 9 10	

Notes

Daily Medication

Date ____/____/____

Medications	Morning	Afternoon	Evening
Drug & Dose:	Time:		
Drug & Dose:			
Drug & Dose:			
Drug & Dose:			
Drug & Dose:			
Drug & Dose:			
Drug & Dose:			

Daily Statistics

Weight:	Temp:	Hours Slept:
Heart rate:	Walking time:	Blood Pressure:
How do you feel ⇨ (1 being poor) circle:	1 2 3 4 5 6 7 8 9 10	

Notes

Daily Medication

Date ____/____/____

Medications	Morning	Afternoon	Evening
Drug & Dose:	Time:		
Drug & Dose:			
Drug & Dose:			
Drug & Dose:			
Drug & Dose:			
Drug & Dose:			
Drug & Dose:			

Daily Statistics

Weight:	Temp:	Hours Slept:
Heart rate:	Walking time:	Blood Pressure:
How do you feel ⇨ (1 being poor) circle:	1 2 3 4 5 6 7 8 9 10	

Notes

Daily Medication

Date ____/____/____

Medications	Morning	Afternoon	Evening
Drug & Dose:	Time:		
Drug & Dose:			
Drug & Dose:			
Drug & Dose:			
Drug & Dose:			
Drug & Dose:			
Drug & Dose:			

Daily Statistics

Weight:	Temp:	Hours Slept:
Heart rate:	Walking time:	Blood Pressure:
How do you feel ⇨ (1 being poor) circle:	1 2 3 4 5 6 7 8 9 10	

Notes

Daily Medication

Date ____/____/____

Medications	Morning	Afternoon	Evening
Drug & Dose:	Time:		
Drug & Dose:			
Drug & Dose:			
Drug & Dose:			
Drug & Dose:			
Drug & Dose:			
Drug & Dose:			

Daily Statistics

Weight:	Temp:	Hours Slept:
Heart rate:	Walking time:	Blood Pressure:
How do you feel ⇨ (1 being poor) circle:	1 2 3 4 5 6 7 8 9 10	

Notes

Daily Medication

Date ____/____/____

Medications	Morning	Afternoon	Evening
Drug & Dose:	Time:		
Drug & Dose:			
Drug & Dose:			
Drug & Dose:			
Drug & Dose:			
Drug & Dose:			
Drug & Dose:			

Daily Statistics

Weight:	Temp:	Hours Slept:
Heart rate:	Walking time:	Blood Pressure:
How do you feel ⇨ (1 being poor) circle:	1 2 3 4 5 6 7 8 9 10	

Notes

Daily Medication

Date ____/____/____

Medications	Morning	Afternoon	Evening
Drug & Dose:	Time:		
Drug & Dose:			
Drug & Dose:			
Drug & Dose:			
Drug & Dose:			
Drug & Dose:			
Drug & Dose:			

Daily Statistics

Weight:	Temp:	Hours Slept:
Heart rate:	Walking time:	Blood Pressure:
How do you feel ⇨ (1 being poor) circle:	1 2 3 4 5 6 7 8 9 10	

Notes

Daily Medication

Date ____/____/____

Medications	Morning	Afternoon	Evening
Drug & Dose:	Time:		
Drug & Dose:			
Drug & Dose:			
Drug & Dose:			
Drug & Dose:			
Drug & Dose:			
Drug & Dose:			

Daily Statistics

Weight:	Temp:	Hours Slept:
Heart rate:	Walking time:	Blood Pressure:
How do you feel ⇨ (1 being poor) circle:	1 2 3 4 5 6 7 8 9 10	

Appointments

2014

January
S	M	T	W	T	F	S
			1	2	3	4
5	6	7	8	9	10	11
12	13	14	15	16	17	18
19	20	21	22	23	24	25
26	27	28	29	30	31	

February
S	M	T	W	T	F	S
						1
2	3	4	5	6	7	8
9	10	11	12	13	14	15
16	17	18	19	20	21	22
23	24	25	26	27	28	

March
S	M	T	W	T	F	S
						1
2	3	4	5	6	7	8
9	10	11	12	13	14	15
16	17	18	19	20	21	22
23	24	25	26	27	28	29
30	31					

April
S	M	T	W	T	F	S
		1	2	3	4	5
6	7	8	9	10	11	12
13	14	15	16	17	18	19
20	21	22	23	24	25	26
27	28	29	30			

May
S	M	T	W	T	F	S
				1	2	3
4	5	6	7	8	9	10
11	12	13	14	15	16	17
18	19	20	21	22	23	24
25	26	27	28	29	30	31

June
S	M	T	W	T	F	S
1	2	3	4	5	6	7
8	9	10	11	12	13	14
15	16	17	18	19	20	21
22	23	24	25	26	27	28
29	30					

July
S	M	T	W	T	F	S
		1	2	3	4	5
6	7	8	9	10	11	12
13	14	15	16	17	18	19
20	21	22	23	24	25	26
27	28	29	30	31		

August
S	M	T	W	T	F	S
					1	2
3	4	5	6	7	8	9
10	11	12	13	14	15	16
17	18	19	20	21	22	23
24	25	26	27	28	29	30
31						

September
S	M	T	W	T	F	S
	1	2	3	4	5	6
7	8	9	10	11	12	13
14	15	16	17	18	19	20
21	22	23	24	25	26	27
28	29	30				

October
S	M	T	W	T	F	S
			1	2	3	4
5	6	7	8	9	10	11
12	13	14	15	16	17	18
19	20	21	22	23	24	25
26	27	28	29	30	31	

November
S	M	T	W	T	F	S
						1
2	3	4	5	6	7	8
9	10	11	12	13	14	15
16	17	18	19	20	21	22
23	24	25	26	27	28	29
30						

December
S	M	T	W	T	F	S
	1	2	3	4	5	6
7	8	9	10	11	12	13
14	15	16	17	18	19	20
21	22	23	24	25	26	27
28	29	30	31			

Appointments

2015

January
S	M	T	W	T	F	S
				1	2	3
4	5	6	7	8	9	10
11	12	13	14	15	16	17
18	19	20	21	22	23	24
25	26	27	28	29	30	31

February
S	M	T	W	T	F	S
1	2	3	4	5	6	7
8	9	10	11	12	13	14
15	16	17	18	19	20	21
22	23	24	25	26	27	28

March
S	M	T	W	T	F	S
1	2	3	4	5	6	7
8	9	10	11	12	13	14
15	16	17	18	19	20	21
22	23	24	25	26	27	28
29	30	31				

April
S	M	T	W	T	F	S
			1	2	3	4
5	6	7	8	9	10	11
12	13	14	15	16	17	18
19	20	21	22	23	24	25
26	27	28	29	30		

May
S	M	T	W	T	F	S
					1	2
3	4	5	6	7	8	9
10	11	12	13	14	15	16
17	18	19	20	21	22	23
24	25	26	27	28	29	30
31						

June
S	M	T	W	T	F	S
	1	2	3	4	5	6
7	8	9	10	11	12	13
14	15	16	17	18	19	20
21	22	23	24	25	26	27
28	29	30				

July
S	M	T	W	T	F	S
			1	2	3	4
5	6	7	8	9	10	11
12	13	14	15	16	17	18
19	20	21	22	23	24	25
26	27	28	29	30	31	

August
S	M	T	W	T	F	S
						1
2	3	4	5	6	7	8
9	10	11	12	13	14	15
16	17	18	19	20	21	22
23	24	25	26	27	28	29
30	31					

September
S	M	T	W	T	F	S
		1	2	3	4	5
6	7	8	9	10	11	12
13	14	15	16	17	18	19
20	21	22	23	24	25	26
27	28	29	30			

October
S	M	T	W	T	F	S
				1	2	3
4	5	6	7	8	9	10
11	12	13	14	15	16	17
18	19	20	21	22	23	24
25	26	27	28	29	30	31

November
S	M	T	W	T	F	S
1	2	3	4	5	6	7
8	9	10	11	12	13	14
15	16	17	18	19	20	21
22	23	24	25	26	27	28
29	30					

December
S	M	T	W	T	F	S
		1	2	3	4	5
6	7	8	9	10	11	12
13	14	15	16	17	18	19
20	21	22	23	24	25	26
27	28	29	30	31		

Appointments

2016

January
S	M	T	W	T	F	S
					1	2
3	4	5	6	7	8	9
10	11	12	13	14	15	16
17	18	19	20	21	22	23
24	25	26	27	28	29	30
31						

February
S	M	T	W	T	F	S
	1	2	3	4	5	6
7	8	9	10	11	12	13
14	15	16	17	18	19	20
21	22	23	24	25	26	27
28	29					

March
S	M	T	W	T	F	S
		1	2	3	4	5
6	7	8	9	10	11	12
13	14	15	16	17	18	19
20	21	22	23	24	25	26
27	28	29	30	31		

April
S	M	T	W	T	F	S
					1	2
3	4	5	6	7	8	9
10	11	12	13	14	15	16
17	18	19	20	21	22	23
24	25	26	27	28	29	30

May
S	M	T	W	T	F	S
1	2	3	4	5	6	7
8	9	10	11	12	13	14
15	16	17	18	19	20	21
22	23	24	25	26	27	28
29	30	31				

June
S	M	T	W	T	F	S
			1	2	3	4
5	6	7	8	9	10	11
12	13	14	15	16	17	18
19	20	21	22	23	24	25
26	27	28	29	30		

July
S	M	T	W	T	F	S
					1	2
3	4	5	6	7	8	9
10	11	12	13	14	15	16
17	18	19	20	21	22	23
24	25	26	27	28	29	30
31						

August
S	M	T	W	T	F	S
	1	2	3	4	5	6
7	8	9	10	11	12	13
14	15	16	17	18	19	20
21	22	23	24	25	26	27
28	29	30	31			

September
S	M	T	W	T	F	S
				1	2	3
4	5	6	7	8	9	10
11	12	13	14	15	16	17
18	19	20	21	22	23	24
25	26	27	28	29	30	

October
S	M	T	W	T	F	S
						1
2	3	4	5	6	7	8
9	10	11	12	13	14	15
16	17	18	19	20	21	22
23	24	25	26	27	28	29
30	31					

November
S	M	T	W	T	F	S
		1	2	3	4	5
6	7	8	9	10	11	12
13	14	15	16	17	18	19
20	21	22	23	24	25	26
27	28	29	30			

December
S	M	T	W	T	F	S
				1	2	3
4	5	6	7	8	9	10
11	12	13	14	15	16	17
18	19	20	21	22	23	24
25	26	27	28	29	30	31

Appointments

2017

January
S	M	T	W	T	F	S
						7
1	2	3	4	5	6	
8	9	10	11	12	13	14
15	16	17	18	19	20	21
22	23	24	25	26	27	28
29	30	31				

February
S	M	T	W	T	F	S
			1	2	3	4
5	6	7	8	9	10	11
12	13	14	15	16	17	18
19	20	21	22	23	24	25
26	27	28				

March
S	M	T	W	T	F	S
			1	2	3	4
5	6	7	8	9	10	11
12	13	14	15	16	17	18
19	20	21	22	23	24	25
26	27	28	29	30	31	

April
S	M	T	W	T	F	S
						1
2	3	4	5	6	7	8
9	10	11	12	13	14	15
16	17	18	19	20	21	22
23	24	25	26	27	28	29
30						

May
S	M	T	W	T	F	S
	1	2	3	4	5	6
7	8	9	10	11	12	13
14	15	16	17	18	19	20
21	22	23	24	25	26	27
28	29	30	31			

June
S	M	T	W	T	F	S
				1	2	3
4	5	6	7	8	9	10
11	12	13	14	15	16	17
18	19	20	21	22	23	24
25	26	27	28	29	30	

July
S	M	T	W	T	F	S
						1
2	3	4	5	6	7	8
9	10	11	12	13	14	15
16	17	18	19	20	21	22
23	24	25	26	27	28	29
30	31					

August
S	M	T	W	T	F	S
		1	2	3	4	5
6	7	8	9	10	11	12
13	14	15	16	17	18	19
20	21	22	23	24	25	26
27	28	29	30	31		

September
S	M	T	W	T	F	S
					1	2
3	4	5	6	7	8	9
10	11	12	13	14	15	16
17	18	19	20	21	22	23
24	25	26	27	28	29	30

October
S	M	T	W	T	F	S
1	2	3	4	5	6	7
8	9	10	11	12	13	14
15	16	17	18	19	20	21
22	23	24	25	26	27	28
29	30	31				

November
S	M	T	W	T	F	S
			1	2	3	4
5	6	7	8	9	10	11
12	13	14	15	16	17	18
19	20	21	22	23	24	25
26	27	28	29	30		

December
S	M	T	W	T	F	S
					1	2
3	4	5	6	7	8	9
10	11	12	13	14	15	16
17	18	19	20	21	22	23
24	25	26	27	28	29	30
31						

Appointments

2018

January
S	M	T	W	T	F	S
	1	2	3	4	5	6
7	8	9	10	11	12	13
14	15	16	17	18	19	20
21	22	23	24	25	26	27
28	29	30	31			

February
S	M	T	W	T	F	S
				1	2	3
4	5	6	7	8	9	10
11	12	13	14	15	16	17
18	19	20	21	22	23	24
25	26	27	28			

March
S	M	T	W	T	F	S
				1	2	3
4	5	6	7	8	9	10
11	12	13	14	15	16	17
18	19	20	21	22	23	24
25	26	27	28	29	30	31

April
S	M	T	W	T	F	S
1	2	3	4	5	6	7
8	9	10	11	12	13	14
15	16	17	18	19	20	21
22	23	24	25	26	27	28
29	30					

May
S	M	T	W	T	F	S
		1	2	3	4	5
6	7	8	9	10	11	12
13	14	15	16	17	18	19
20	21	22	23	24	25	26
27	28	29	30	31		

June
S	M	T	W	T	F	S
					1	2
3	4	5	6	7	8	9
10	11	12	13	14	15	16
17	18	19	20	21	22	23
24	25	26	27	28	29	30

July
S	M	T	W	T	F	S
1	2	3	4	5	6	7
8	9	10	11	12	13	14
15	16	17	18	19	20	21
22	23	24	25	26	27	28
29	30	31				

August
S	M	T	W	T	F	S
			1	2	3	4
5	6	7	8	9	10	11
12	13	14	15	16	17	18
19	20	21	22	23	24	25
26	27	28	29	30	31	

September
S	M	T	W	T	F	S
						1
2	3	4	5	6	7	8
9	10	11	12	13	14	15
16	17	18	19	20	21	22
23	24	25	26	27	28	29
30						

October
S	M	T	W	T	F	S
	1	2	3	4	5	6
7	8	9	10	11	12	13
14	15	16	17	18	19	20
21	22	23	24	25	26	27
28	29	30	31			

November
S	M	T	W	T	F	S
				1	2	3
4	5	6	7	8	9	10
11	12	13	14	15	16	17
18	19	20	21	22	23	24
25	26	27	28	29	30	

December
S	M	T	W	T	F	S
						1
2	3	4	5	6	7	8
9	10	11	12	13	14	15
16	17	18	19	20	21	22
23	24	25	26	27	28	29
30	31					

www.ingramcontent.com/pod-product-compliance
Lightning Source LLC
Chambersburg PA
CBHW081143170526
45165CB00008B/2784